Measuring the Effectiveness of Nurse Education:

The Use of Performance Indicators

Central Health Studies:

The Central Health Studies (CHS) series is designed to provide nurses and other health-care professionals with up-to-date, informative texts on key professional and management issues and human skills in health care.

The Consulting Editor:

The series was conceived by John Tingle, BA Law Hons, Cert Ed, M Ed, Barrister, Senior Lecturer in Law, Nottingham Law School, Nottingham Polytechnic. John has published widely on the subject of the professional and legal accountability of health-care professionals.

Central Health Studies is a joint venture between **Quay Publishing Ltd.**, Lancaster and **BKT Information Services**, Nottingham

Central Health Studies
Consulting Editor: John Tingle

Measuring the Effectiveness of Nurse Education:

The Use of Performance Indicators

Aru Narayanasamy

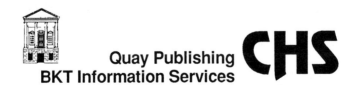

Quay Publishing
BKT Information Services

Quay Publishing Ltd
7.1.9 Cameron House
White Cross, Lancaster LA1 4XQ

ISBN   1-85642-059-0

British Library Cataloguing-in-Publication Data

A catalogue record for this book is available from the British Library.

Designed and typeset by **BKT Information Services**, Nottingham, Specialists in Desktop Publishing, Database Development, and Electronic Media Publishing.

Printed in the United Kingdom by Bell and Bain Ltd., Glasgow

CONTENTS

ACKNOWLEDGEMENT

I am grateful to the following publishers for allowing me to adapt materials from their publications for my book: Further Education Unit, London, *Towards an Educational Audit.* (material for Chapter 7); King Edward Hospital for London *Effective Unit Management.* I. Wickings (Ed.) 1983 (Black Box Model); Society for Research Into Higher Education Ltd., University of Surrey, *Indicators of Performance.* D. Billings (Ed.) 1980 (The Eight Scale Dimension of the Learning Environment and material on Structure, Process and Outcome).

Every effort has been made to trace copyright holders, but if any have been overlooked, the publishers of this book will be pleased to make the necessary arrangements at the earliest opportunity.

Preface

The search for information on measures of performance is, in my experience, like taking a trip around the galaxy and returning with a sense of mystery regarding what it is all about. I drew this conclusion from my earlier studies into the application of performance indicators in nursing education, because the literature on the field is very limited and there is no suitable guide to their application in nurse education. I believe, however, that the success of nurse education depends on the effective use of performance indicators.

Colleges of nursing, midwifery, and health studies are public institutions and, as such, must remain accountable to the public and to fund providers. To meet this requirement, colleges can adopt performance indicators to establish their effectiveness. In order to use performance indicators, managers and staff need a clear indication of the indicators and their effectiveness. This book aims to offer readers a guide to the many facets related to the measurement of performance in nurse education, from students to senior management. The book is essentially a practical guide, but aims also to be informative and authoritative. The many features of performance related to nurse education are identified and appropriate measures are explored.

Early chapters concentrate on clarification of concepts related to performance measures, including definitions, properties and models of performance indicators. Chapters Four and Five are devoted to the application of performance indicators specifically to nurse education. Chapter Five invites the reader to consider the application of some of the less well-known indicators (established in other, more traditional, institutions of higher education) in relation to colleges of nursing, midwifery, and health studies. In addition, a section is included on the introduction of performance indicators into colleges.

Chapter Six gives practical examples of audit forms and tools for the application of performance indicators. Also, readers are offered examples of a range of indicators related to the various aspects of colleges of nursing, midwifery, and health studies. Finally, Chapter Seven draws some conclusions.

Wishing you an enjoyable trip.

Aru Narayanasamy
College Co-ordinator
Mid-Trent College of Nursing and Midwifery
Queens Medical Centre
University Hospital, Nottingham

Chapter One:
What are Performance Indicators?

Case Illustration

Mrs Mary Green is the newly appointed Principal of New College of Nursing and Midwifery, which has several academic departments and a central unit for administration. The college offers a range of courses from certificate to degree level. Mary is required to produce a report on the performance of her college to the Board of Governors. She is keen to develop a comprehensive set of performance indicators (PIs) to evaluate the effectiveness of her college, so that she can use the information to write the report.

Mary feels instinctively that her college is performing well, is cost-effective in its use of resources, has high standards of teaching and morale, and will score highly in any comparison with other similar establishments. How does she prove this to the Board of Governors?

Introduction

Colleges of Nursing, Midwifery and Health Studies, as public services, are required to be efficient and cost-effective. This means that colleges have to take great care to maintain high standards and to be able to give an account to others of their functions and achievements.

How can we prove to outsiders that a college is 'efficient' and operates in a cost-effective manner? How do we measure such nebulous attributes as the 'viability of teaching methods' or 'staff satisfaction'? The most obvious way is to provide series of data which illustrate performance and can be compared with similar data from other institutions. To do this we need to choose a series of criteria which can be measured easily. These are our 'performance indicators'. We then need to introduce systems into the organisation whereby suitable data can be collected, analysed and presented concisely in the form of a report. This book sets out to examine the range of performance indicators useful in colleges for healthcare professionals and to show how they can be developed and used.

Although, the interest in Performance Indicators (PIs) is not new to the National Health Service (NHS), there is an acute need for a concise practical book such as this one. Since 1987, when new management techniques were adopted, managers concerned about the performance of their organisation within the NHS have been aware of PIs as tools of management. PIs were developed by expert committees which included members from the NHS operational levels. There are several sets of PIs for acute care, for mental health, old people, children, estate management, manpower and so on. One of my recent studies suggests that there is ample scope in nurse education for the development of PIs as measures of institutional performance (Narayanasamy, 1991).

To be able to apply performance indicators, managers must:

- understand what they are;
- be aware of their range and scope;
- choose a set of indicators that will generate the data required;
- set up systems to introduce these measures into the organisation; and
- collect and analyse data on an ongoing basis.

Before continuing with your reading, consider the example given at the beginning of the chapter and attempt the following activities:

Activity one: Define what you mean by 'Performance Indicators'.

Activity two: Which aspects of her college do you think that Mary should be evaluating for effectiveness?

Feedback on Activities: The following sections introduce PIs and outline the aspects of organisations where PIs are necessary for the evaluation of effectiveness.

What are Performance Indicators?

'Performance' means an execution of a function, and this applies to both organisations and human functions. 'Indicator' simply means 'pointer'. PIs can be defined as pointers which focus attention on functions such as resource use, quality of services, staff performance, support services, etc. The RCN (1987) regards PIs as an important management tool and thus define these as 'tools developed to measure and indicate efficiency and effectiveness of an organisation', whilst, Evans (1987, p. 7) defines PIs as:

2

"... a tool which may be used by managers or in our case by educationalists to review and explore systems and processes, and to assess results"

There is a consensus in these definitions that PIs are valuable as tools of institutional measurement. In nurse education, for example, PIs include measures related to :

- Organisation and Management
- Staff Performance
- Teaching Methods
- Learning Environment
- Unit Costs
- Student/Staff Ratio (SSRs)
- Wastage and Completion Rates
- Value Added Scores
- Examination/Assessment Results

As an example, let us consider ways of illustrating how well or how badly a college is doing in terms of staff performance. The following table gives questions that might be asked and a series of indicators that might be used in answering them.

Staff performance

Academic Leadership
Are managers exercising appropriate leadership and ensuring that programmes are relevant to the demands of the market (caring and other services) they serve?

Questions	Performance Indicators
What evidence is there for academic leadership in the institution?	Record of outcome of course
	• No. of new submissions
	• No. of new developments introduced
	• Nature of liaison with validating bodies
	• Extent of staff development, e.g. courses completed; research; consultancy; updating for senior staff

- National/Regional links and relationships

- Evidence of cost-effectiveness of developmental activity

To what extent are institutional managers undertaking effective individual/team development?

- Course team development

- Subject specialist development

- Individual staff development

- Availability of managers to their teams

- Conscious activities to ensure high morale

Types of Indicator

We can distinguish three types of indicator: simple indicators, performance indicators, and general indicators.

Simple Indicators

These are usually expressed as absolute figures and are intended to provide a relatively impartial description of a situation or process. Management statistics (statistical information) are one example of these that you will come across. Simple Indicators are more or less neutral indicators. In other words, these are factual items of information which are interpreted in order to make informed decisions. An example is provided below:

Examination Results 1992 (Registered General Nursing Course)

Date	Numbers		Percentage	
	Entered	Passes	Pass	National
January	16	16	100	85.2
May	15	15	100	83.2
July	45	45	100	83.3
Total	76	76	100	

Activity three: List some types of statistical data that fall into the category of simple indicators.

Performance Indicators (PIs)

These include a standard, an objective, an assessment, or a comparator, and are therefore relative rather than absolute in character. Some simple indicators may become PIs if a value judgement is involved.

Activity four: Imagine you are required to evaluate your courses for effectiveness in terms of teaching methods. List some examples of questions and indicators that you might use in carrying out such an evaluation.

Some examples of PIs related to teaching methods are given below:

Teaching Methods
Are courses evaluated for effectiveness in terms of teaching methods?

Questions	Performance Indicators
Are there opportunities and support for staff to experience different teaching styles?	• Student evaluation/Feedback
Is there evidence of a variety of teaching skills demonstrated by all teaching staff?	• As above • Classroom visits • Peer review feedback • Documentation

What are Performance Indicators?

General Indicators

Opinions, survey findings or general statistics can be regarded as General Indicators. General Indicators can be converted into legitimate PIs. Opinion surveys could be used to determine consumer satisfaction (e.g. student satisfaction with staff) and the findings could be expressed in terms of general statistics (e.g. 60% very satisfied, 20% satisfied, 20% not satisfied). These then become performance indicators, forming part of the overall staff review, as shown below:

Learning Environment
How effective is the learning environment?

Questions	Performance Indicators
Is the climate suggestive of staff and student satisfaction?	• Consumer/staff satisfaction survey questionnaires
	• Quality of staff/student interaction
How effective is the clinical learning environment?	• Availability of profiles of placement
	• Audit tools used
	• Regularity of auditing
	• Review of completed audits
	• Decisions regarding suitability of placement as a learning area taken and communicated?
Is there evidence of peer evaluation of the learning environment?	• Peer evaluation review feedback
	• Teamwork

It is important to realise that PIs are only tools—an aid to the organisation's management—and therefore must be regarded as such. They are not recipes for measurements of all aspects of an organisation. PIs must be treated as signals or guides rather than absolute measures since indicators do not necessarily offer direct measurements of things like resources (inputs), teaching (processes) and successes/failures (outputs).

Advantages of Performance Indicators

The application of PI measures leads to several advantages to the organisation.

Performance indicators:

1. Measure and indicate efficiency and effectiveness of organisation.

2. Are resources which help managers to determine whether a service is efficient and effective by comparison with a given goal.

3. Give, if properly used, a comprehensive and objective view of organisational effectiveness.

4. Allow organisation to thrive, as troubleshooting can take place periodically.

Summary

Colleges of Nursing, Midwifery and Health Studies, as complex corporate organisations, must remain accountable to the public and fund providers in terms of their effectiveness. Performance indicators have potential as performance measures and offer opportunities for educational institutions to monitor their standards. There are subtle differences between types of indicators loosely defined as simple, performance, and general indicators. The emerging evidence suggests that there is scope for developing PIs related to staff performance, teaching methods, learning environment, student-staff ratio (SSR), unit costs, wastage rates, and value-added for colleges of nursing (Narayanasamy, 1991). Having chosen our performance indicators, it is important that they satisfy the criteria of **reliability** and **validity**. The next chapter deals with such properties of performance indicators.

Chapter Two:
Properties of Performance Indicators

The evaluation of the performance of an organisation must involve the assessment of people's attitudes, feelings, and impressions. Questionnaires are useful for recording attitudes relating to organisations, but feelings and impressions are hard to measure: qualitative interpretation of data must be relied on. Accurate reporting of these findings eliminates any distortion of facts and adds to the objectivity of data. Qualitative reports can be used to substantiate findings related to other, more concrete, data. Interpretation of qualitative data involves subjective analysis and explanation of information obtained from questionnaires, interviews, etc. All the procedures used for obtaining data must be **reliable** and **valid**.

Activity: What do you mean by '*validity*' and '*reliability*'?

Validity

The following are ways in which a measure can be considered in terms of validity.

Face Validity

A measure or procedure has face validity when it appears to measure that which it was designed to measure. Face validity is concerned with whether a measure 'looks' right and meets public-relations criteria.

Criterion-related validity

This relates to how well a measure compares with other measures claiming to measure similar items, and how it works practically in a given situation. Does the measure discriminate adequately between problem aspects of an organisation and satisfactory aspects?

Construct-related validity

This relates to how well a measure corresponds to theoretical predictions regarding a given situation. Measures which agree well with theoretical prediction are said to have a high construct-related validity.

9

Content validity

Does the procedure cover a representative sample of the behaviour that is to be measured? For example, if you want to evaluate teaching methods, does the evaluation procedure cover most of the aspects of teaching?

Predictive validity

A procedure has predictive validity if measures obtained can be used to make an accurate prediction of future performance.

Reliability

Reliable indicators produce consistent results whenever performance is evaluated using them. A measure can be considered reliable if:

- different people using the same indicators to measure the same thing obtain similar results; and
- the same person using the same indicator obtains similar results on several occasions.

Characteristics of Performance Indicators

To ensure that your PIs are valid and reliable, you may carry out several pilot studies using some of the ideas and examples provided in this book. Pilot measurements act as a test for ensuring reliability and validity. If the pilot PIs do not measure-up in terms of validity and reliability, then some of the indicators may need re-shaping.

Furthermore, PIs must not be misinterpreted and must certainly be free from both statistical and personal bias. Statistical bias is a product of inappropriate techniques of measurement, and personal bias is a product of conscious manipulation of information for personal gain. It is not unusual for PIs to be subjected to personal bias to adapt their interpretation to organisational fit. PIs should be cheat-proof: if they are not, institutions will only be cheating themselves.

The characteristics of good performance indicators are: availability, awareness, accessibility, extensiveness, appropriateness, efficiency, effectiveness, outcome, benefits/impacts, and acceptability (Sizer, 1979). Sizer's table of properties of PIs is given below.

Properties of Performance Indicators
(Source: Sizer, 1979, pp. 58)

Focus of Measure	Conceptual Content	Tells
Availability	Amount and type of course, research, facility, or central services.	What can be obtained.
Examples: List of services in Careers Advisors Service; list of research facilities and opportunities available in academic department; number, capacities and location of lecture and seminar rooms.		

Focus of Measure	Conceptual Content	Tells
Awareness	Knowledge of user population of existence, range and conditions for entry or use of courses, research facilities, or central services.	Who knows about what is available.
Examples: Knowledge of prospective students of course offered by an academic department. Knowledge by prospective user of services provided by central computer centre.		

Focus of Measure	Conceptual Content	Tells
Accessibility	Indicates if services can be obtained.	Ease of reaching and using facility.
Examples: Availability of photocopying facilities: location of car parks; average waiting time for literature search by library/information service; opening hours of medical centre.		

Focus of Measure	Conceptual Content	Tells
Extensiveness	Compare quantity of services rendered with capacity available and/or potential demand	'How much' but not 'How well'

Examples:
Students enrolled on course against course quotas: number of users in library: clients in medical centre: percentage of final-year students using careers advisory service: utilisation of lecture and seminar rooms

Focus of Measure	Conceptual Content	Tells
Efficiency	Compare resources inputs with outputs	Quantity of resource utilisation: –How much did it cost per unit –How much did it cost in total –How much did it take –What grade of employee was used

Examples:
Cost per client service in medical centre: cost per student by course: cost per literature search: cost per meal served

Focus of Measure	Conceptual Content	Tells
Effectiveness	Compares accomplishments with objectives –Qualitative –Comparative	Characteristics –Duration –Content Effect –Proportion served –Variance from budget standards

Examples:
Comparison of planned with actual: utilisation of lecture and seminar rooms: number of students graduating: number of graduates employed: ratio of actual utilisation to planned utilisation of computer: comparison of budgets cost of central service with actual cost: comparison of actual cost per FTE for course with planned: comparison of planned course content with actual course content: actual wastage rate compared with planned wastage rate.

Focus of Measure	Conceptual Content	Tells
Outcome/benefits/ impacts	Identifies social or economic benefits	Monetary effects Non-monetary effects

Examples:
Increase in earnings arising from attendance at/graduation from course: benefits to society from successful research into previously incurable disease: patents and copyrights registered

Focus of Measure	Conceptual Content	Tells
Acceptability	Access match of service/course/ research outcome with user participant preferences	User satisfaction with services. Student satisfaction with courses. Client satisfaction with outcome of sponsored research.

Examples:
Demand for courses: number of complaints to libraries: course evaluation at end of lecture programme: repeat sponsorship of research

Before you use any of these PIs you must ensure that they are relevant, accurate and feasible for your institution. Relevance implies that the indicator measures something which is important for the effective management of the institution. The accuracy of PIs in measuring true underlying performance, relative to the organisation's given objectives is important. Economic feasibility is another important aspect of PIs. Does the benefit of producing the PI outweigh the costs incurred, particularly at the margin?

Furthermore, in order that PIs are absolutely appropriate, you must ensure that individuals participating in organisational measurements, although working independently, develop essentially similar measures or conclusions from an examination of the same evidence or data.

Finally, PIs must be institutionally acceptable, in that it is vital that the people using the indicators should accept them as relevant and fair. Also, PIs must be neutral in the political and behavioural sense. By political neutrality, I mean that the process of collecting and using the indicator should not undesirably distort patterns of power and influence either within the organisation or between organisation and external parties. As to behavioural neutrality, I mean that the actual process of collecting and using the indicator should not distort undesirably the behaviour of individuals or groups within the organisation. In the next chapter, models of performance indicators will be considered.

Further Activities

1. Try to construct some PIs for measuring teaching effectiveness. Do these contain the properties of PIs as advanced by Sizer?

2. How would you ensure that these indicators are reliable and valid?

Chapter Three:
Models of Performance Indicators

Models can provide a useful framework for developing a set of performance indicators to measure the attributes of an organisation. In this chapter, I consider several models that can be applied in the field of nurse education.

Activity: Define what you mean by a model.

The word 'model' is frequently used in everyday language. Technically, a model is a conceptual representation of a reality. It can be a symbolic or an abstract representation of a real thing. For example, a miniature model car is a representation of a real car. On the other hand, an abstract model is difficult to assemble in the physical sense although it is not too difficult to demonstrate in diagrammatic form. A model (symbolic or abstract) helps us to simplify reality and thus aids understanding of complex situations. Models of PIs fall into the 'abstract' category.

No one model can be used in isolation when an institution's performance is being evaluated. The varied nature and purpose of PIs does not fit into a particular framework which can be conveniently defined in terms of a particular model. Several conceptual models may be necessary to assess a complex institution such as a higher education establishment to get the best out of PIs. An eclectic use of models is the way forward for institutional performance measurement. Some models suitable for PIs are discussed below.

Inputs and Outputs Model

The Inputs and Outputs model lends itself well to performance measurements. It is a simplified conceptual framework which views higher education as a process. This process transforms input into outputs, and is itself part of wider economic and social process.

Figure 1 provides us with a symbolic representation of a reality in an abstract form. In this model, higher education is viewed as a process for transforming inputs (human and material resources) into either teaching or research outputs.

Outputs include the value-added of those receiving instruction from a college or other higher education institution: undergraduate students, graduate students, and those taking short courses. Outputs also include any increment in the knowledge of students, whether or not they complete their studies. Some outputs are direct as consumer benefits, for example, a mastery of a discipline or completion of research may yield direct satisfaction.

Figure 1:   Inputs and Outputs Model

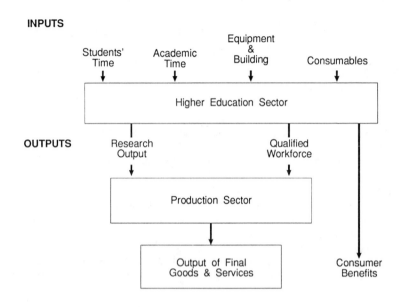

How does this model fit in with performance measures related to, for example, a College of Nursing, Midwifery and Health Studies? Let us take Staff Performance as an example to answer this question.

Staff Development	
Input PIs	**Outcome PIs**
Effectiveness of: –course team development –subject specialist development –individual staff development –availability of managers to their teams	What are the benefits? –staff motivation –staff expertise –role relationships –staff satisfaction with development programmes

Other output measures related to staff development may include:

Context	PIs
Staff satisfaction	Records of staff meetings, interviews, counselling
Provision of staff development opportunities	Staff development policy statement; staff development programme; records of in-service development programme activities; records of counselling meetings
Evaluation of staff development	Records of evaluation procedures; questionnaires

Further examples are given in Chapter Six.

When using the input/output model we should consider other factors which affect the performance outcome of an institution. These factors may be, for example, unobservable situations and constraints. In order to consider these factors, especially in complex organisations such as the National Health Service, Best (1983) proposes a 'Black Box' model.

Figure 2:   Black Box model of complex System

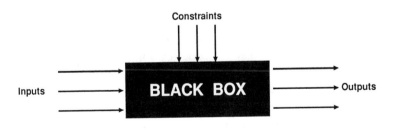

Source: Best (1983) p. 65.

17

Best (p. 65) explains this model thus:

> "Typically, systems investigated in this manner have
> been 'unobservable' in the sense there is no possibility
> of constructing a causal explanation of their behaviour
> through observation of their 'inner' workings. Hence
> the term 'black (that is, opaque) box' "

The black box gives us a framework in which the analysis must proceed on the basis of observation and measurement of whatever features of the system the external observer may be able to detect. The implication of this model is particularly useful in an institution, such as the NHS, where it is not clearly understood how inputs are transformed into outputs. The black box model adds another dimension to the input/output model introduced earlier. It highlights the importance of paying close attention to certain unobservable or hidden factors in the analysis of PIs in an institution. For instance, where we find great discrepancy between input and output (for example, low resources but high-quality results), we must look closely at what factors may be involved regardless of the complexity of the system.

Structure–Process–Outcome Model (Donabedian, 1966)

This model has been discussed in relation to nurse education (Kershaw and Evans, 1986; RCN, 1987 & 1988). The terms structure, process, and outcome are defined as follows:

Structure: the working environment of the system under review, including organisational and management characteristics, physical facilities/equipment, staff work patterns, grades of staff, specialist qualifications and education, and aspects decided upon internally or 'imposed'.

Process: a series of actions, changes or functions that brings about an end or result.

Outcome: the results to be achieved.

The RCN's examples for developing PIs using this model are given below.

Standard statements	Structure	Process	Outcome
Standard requirement	Consider the system by which the standard is to be achieved.	Review the process by which the standard is achieved.	Measure the outcome in relation to the standard set.

Definition of standard

A standard is defined as:

> "a yardstick consisting of a specific set of factors, relating to a particular entity, which may be in the form of a specification or a measurement of quality, cost, performance, manufacturing, etc."

Anderson, 1983, p. 107

In a practical sense, it is an agreed level of service required for a particular purpose. Standards should be reasonable, explicit, useful, measurable, observable and achievable. When we set standards for institutional performance (nurse/midwifery/health studies) it is imperative that we involve teachers, managers, practitioners, consumers (students) and purchasers (contract parties) so that they all can get an explicit view of the process and practice of education by being a party to decisions about standards setting. If you are in the process of setting standards for your organisation, you may consider the following points, as they offer a reliable basis for developing a sound institutional performance procedure.

Standard statements offer the following benefits:

- They reflect values and beliefs about people (e.g. patients, teachers, students, nursing staff), their care, work environment and learning experience.
- They utilise research findings or may identify areas where research is needed in relation to standards/quality statements.
- They act as standards of quality which serve as models to facilitate and evaluate structures, process, and outcomes within/of an educational institution.

Source: RCN, 1987

We have already defined a standard and the benefits to be derived from it. The RCN model can be used for developing PIs in terms of standard statements. The RCN's guidance is clear and well structured, and makes a complex procedure relatively easy to follow. I suggest the following steps when developing a Performance Indicator model for your institution.

i.   Set standards

ii.   Ask questions related to the standards using the Structure-Process-Outcome model.

iii. Identify the arising educational PIs.

'Arising PIs' is a term used to embrace the indicators which are identified as a result of asking questions using the Structure-Process-Outcome format in an institution. A model for developing 'Arising Educational PIs' is given in Figure 3.

Figure 3: A Model for Developing 'Arising Educational Performance Indicators'

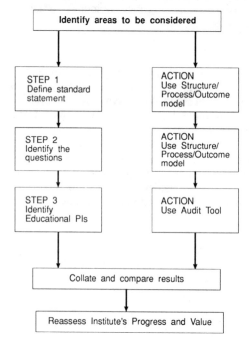

Source: RCN (1988) p 9.

Summary

The RCN's proposition is valuable and practical in that it meets the four requirements of a model advocated by Glazer and Strauss (1967):

1. It is closely related and applied to the daily realities of the area in which it is to be used.

2. It is understandable to the people using it.

3. It is general enough to cover the ever-changing practice situations, yet concrete enough to be relevant to and account for everyday situations.

4. It enables the user of the theory (practitioner) to have enough control over the everyday situation to make its application productive.

However, in spite of the ability to meet the above criteria, the RCN's Structure–Process–Outcome model has a serious drawback. It is cumbersome and requires time to sort out where the probing questions/PIs should be placed, i.e., whether under the headings of Structure or Process or Outcome. However, do not be put off by this initial difficulty, as with some perseverance it becomes less difficult to fit PIs into appropriate categories. At the end of this exercise, i.e. sorting PIs under these headings, you should have a reasonable set of PIs for your institution. An example of PIs under the headings of Structure, Process and Outcome is given below.

Standard Statement	Structure	Process	Outcome
Students have a right to receive supervision and support from an identified, qualified nurse who facilitates the student's development	Each Student has an identified mentor. Selection of the mentor should be negotiable between both parties. There is commitment to developing the mentor system. Mentors should be suitably prepared to undertake their task. Students' practice is supervised.	Opportunities are given to qualified staff to prepare them for the mentor role. Mentors have an active involvement with their students. On-duty rotas should reflect the need to allow the student and mentor to work together	Students can expect to work with their mentor on at least 2 spans of duty per week. Mentors actively teach and supervise their students. Students have an opportunity to participate in selecting their mentor.
Arising Performance Indicators	1. Students have a named mentor identified. 2. Mentors supervise the work of their students on a regular basis. 3. Mentors are involved in the assessment of their named students. 4. The mentor system is effective in providing support for the student. 5. Mentors should have no more than two students to supervise at any one time.		

Source: RCN (1988) p. 14

Cybernetic Model

Finally, I suggest the Cybernetic Model (Figure 4) for applying PIs as a measure of your organisation's effectiveness. This model is one in which information relating to performance is compared against a performance standard (see illustration, next page). The idea of this model (developed by Sproull and Zubrow, 1981) is one based on the cybernetic model which employs the analogy of a thermostat. They state:

> "The model suggests that when information indicates the organisation is performing poorly, corrective action is taken to bring organisation performance back into line. Information is collected and used to improve performance."

Sproull and Zubrow (1981) p. 67

Figure 4:   A True Cybernetic System

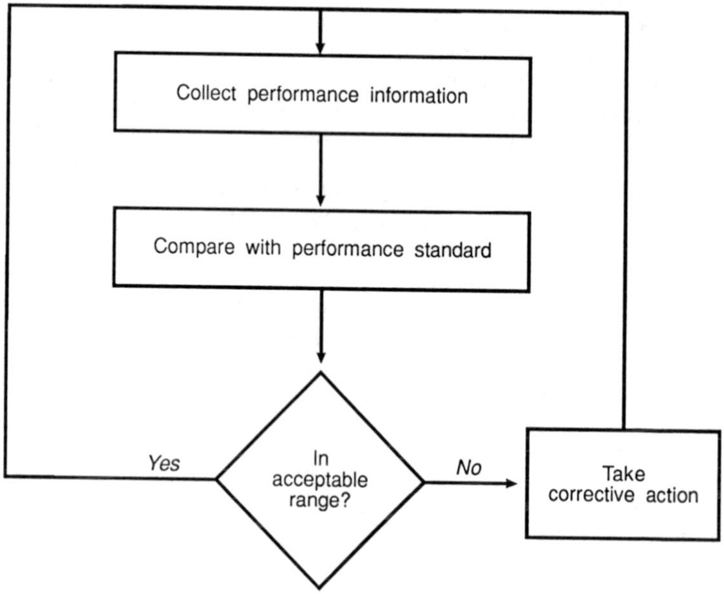

Source: Sproull & Zubrow (1981) p 69.

The illustration above depicts the nature of this feedback system. This model spells out the common rationales for management information system and management by objectives. Some questions and indicators pertaining to management information systems are given on p54–56.

Also, it underlines concerns about the use of evaluation information in a social programme. In a true cybernetic system, information is used to indicate adequate performance as well an inadequate performance. Below, I give an example to demonstrate the application of this model to an academic audit process for the Project 2000 Course in a College of Nursing and Midwifery.

A Model For Actioning Academic Auditing

The example below indicates that the Cybernetic Model is a practical one. It offers a lot of scope for comprehensive examination of an institution's performance in terms of indicators and emphasises that the results must be interpreted before conclusions are drawn.

Figure 5: Application of the Cybernetic Model

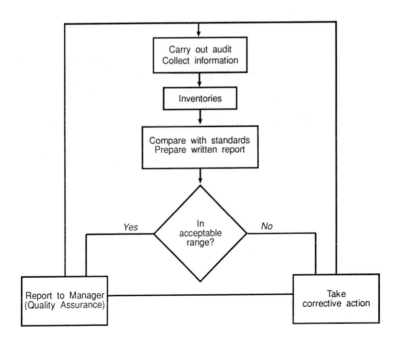

The Cybernetic Model guides you as to what you can do with the information. However, a note of caution concerning this model: you must consider the three factors highlighted below:

1. Information use should be equated with taking corrective action.

2. Information users should not be equated with information procedures or collection.

3. It should be assumed that information must carry with it implicit strategies for corrective action.

Summary

In this chapter, four sound models for developing educational PIs were introduced and the reasons as to the suitability of each of them as a model for PIs were considered. I recommend that an eclectic approach is the way to make the best use of the various ideas outlined in this chapter. A criterion test of a model for your institution is indicated here, and in the next chapter we will consider the application of PIs to nurse education.

Further Activities

1. Using the Structure–Process–Outcome model, devise some performance indicators for evaluating the effectiveness of the learning environment.

2. What difficulties did you encounter when using the above model? (If you do encounter difficulties, and would like to discuss them with the author, he may be contacted at Mid-Trent College, Queen's Medical Centre, Nottingham.)

3. Using the Cybernetic Model, devise a protocol for an academic audit.

Chapter Four:
Qualitative Factors in Nurse Education

A comprehensive set of PIs is required for nurse education institutions in order to measure their effectiveness. In order to be comprehensive in their evaluation of performance, educational organisations must include indicators related to:

- Management and Organisation;
- Teaching Methods;
- Staff Performance;
- Learning Environment;

} Qualitative Aspects

- Unit Costs;
- Student Staff Ratios (SSR);
- Wastage and Completion Rates;
- Value-added;
- Test Scores/Examinations.

} Quantitative Aspects

We will deal with indicators related to management and organisations, staff performance, teaching methods and learning environment in this chapter and the remaining indicators in the next chapter. Below, I introduce you to some examples of PIs for each of these aspects of nurse education and outline reasons for their use.

Management and Organisation

Performance indicators of organisational management include measures related to the organisation's purpose or mission; organisation strategies; functional areas of management/organisational structure; marketing; decision making and information systems; income-generation activities; and recruitment and selection.

A mission statement spells out the purpose of an institution and succinctly embraces its goals and direction. The purpose or mission statements direct the operational activities of an institution and, more specifically, each of its functional components.

Marketing is a process in which supply is matched with demand, that is, having the right goods or services, of the right quality, in the right place, at the right time, and in the right amounts. Marketing must meet three requirements. Firstly, it must respond to customers' needs; secondly, it must have the organisational processes to respond to customers' demands;

25

and thirdly, it must allow profit making for services given or goods delivered as a result of a mutually agreed contract.

All marketing strategies must reflect dynamic and proactive actions related to the institution's relative position in the market concerning its courses. PIs related to these action strategies will reflect its effectiveness in terms of marketing strategies. The next strategy, though closely related to marketing, but not necessarily part of it, is income-generation activities.

Income-generation strategies must also be clearly defined and demonstrated by actual and potential capacity to bring in income at a profitable level in terms of resource input. The administrative and support mechanisms for income generation should be evaluated for their effectiveness.

A clear and effective system related to decision taking and information is a necessity for an effective institution. The existence of well-defined operational policies makes the job of delegating responsibilities for decision making to the lowest appropriate level much easier and more effective. Decision making must be supported by a comprehensive relevant and up-to-date information system.

A well-defined policy for recruitment and selection is necessary for the institution to be effective. There must be a procedure for measuring agreed standards related to this policy.

Staff Performance

Staff-related PIs offer evaluative measures of the management of human resources and, in particular, management of both teaching and non-teaching staff. The management of education institutions, therefore, consists in large measure of ensuring the most effective and efficient deployment of human resources available. Effective management of teaching staff must be directed, therefore, at achieving the highest possible quality of teaching. Also, staff-related PIs give an overall picture of staff performance in an educational institution which is being evaluated for its effectiveness. Furthermore, an important indicator of staff performance is 'all teaching and research staff's review of their attitudes to course, and, by implication, their roles' (Bethel, 1980). This particular PI would reveal for example the institution's role in, and commitment to, achieving education and staff development. Finally, staff-related indicators would point out whether the objectives of management are met.

In one nurse education institution the following criteria related to staff performance were used successfully:

Staff-related criteria

- accessibility of the Senior Education Manager.
- regular meetings held within:
  a) Department
  b) Team.

- good communication between line managerial post and tutorial staff.
- open discussion periods for staff.
- reading research.
- opportunities for further/higher education.
- funding and study leave.
- provision to replace staff on study leave.

Rogues, 1988

Rogues claims that these criteria, which I consider to be PIs, had enabled her institution to assess the effectiveness and quality of education. In that particular institution, staff were able to go beyond the use of statistical information such as numbers in training, examination results, and wastage —they were successful in producing a tool that was adaptable for accurate evaluation of the education process.

However, the use of indicators related to staff performance must extend beyond academic personnel and include the following:

- continuing education
- staff development
- role of student services (student counselling and welfare, student accommodation, careers and appointments)
- non-academic staff role.

Example One: An institution used performance indicators related to staff development and continuing education. The effectiveness of staff development was revealed by findings of indicators related to staff as follows: there was a significant increase in staff use of Educational Centre's Tutors self-evaluation questionnaires, its student feedback questionnaires, and library's self-directed study facilities.

Example Two: Another institution uses PIs related to student reviews and derives useful information on the following: the academic performance of certain kinds of students; their residential accommodation; and the effects of a placement on students with particular psychological traits. This information is important to course/personal tutors and curriculum developers. The institution can use every factor from the findings to formulate a strategy to improve the performance of the individual student and, cumulatively, of the institution.

Example Three: A third institution has an agreed criterion for promotion of staff and uses a procedure which involves the documentation of the activities of all staff under indicators of performance headings. In this particular institution such indicators included for teaching staff are:

Qualitative Aspects

- subject knowledge and scholarship
- teaching activities
- course tutorship
- contribution to external relationship and commitment to the institution.

It is likely that these indicators would reveal the effectiveness of the institution's staff development policy. This approach is particularly useful for Colleges which are considering a policy for staff promotion.

Finally, when PIs related to staff performance are used, it is important that all staff feel secure in the knowledge that indicators of performance are just, appropriate, and equitable, and that the system is designed to assist them in meeting their targets.

Non-academic staff

It is paramount to recognise the role of non-academic staff in contributing to institutional performance. They also need to be included in the communication/consultation system and to benefit from incentives.

Staff Professional Profile

The staff professional profile (SPP) can be a useful form of performance indicator when an organisational review is carried out with the aim of improving institutional performance. This method can be productive if it is carried out in a systematic manner. It can lead to the identification of problems that hinder the achievement of the organisational missions, so that ways can be found to overcome them. One particular area is the utilisation and development of staff.

An institution can utilise the following as a Staff Professional Profile:

- Assigned teaching profile.
- Professional service to industry/commerce/community.
  a) consultancy
  b) resource applied to specific problem
  c) other professional service.

Benefits of SPP

1. A more effective utilisation of the human resources available to the organisation becomes apparent.

2. The problem of workload equity can be better handled.

3. Teaching assignments are a matter of public record and are determined on a basis of matching needs with available skills across the institution.

4. Personal impediments to improved performance can be identified and discussed in a structurally less threatening situation, and agreed corrective actions can be determined.

5. The need to develop, implement and review a comprehensive staff development scheme is highlighted and some modifications to the future directions of that programme can be determined.

Student Reports

Student reports are useful indicators of teaching staff performance. The results of student reports provide the basis for instructional improvement and decision making. Student reports can justifiably be described as indicators of student (consumer) satisfaction, but their measures as a basis for better staff performance or personal decision should be treated cautiously because of their subjectivity.

Staff Appraisal

Staff-related PIs are closely associated with staff appraisal procedures in that these measures provide information for the managers to help the staff maximise their potentials. Staff-related measures fit in with McGregor's (1960) list of objectives of performance appraisal.

1. **Administrative**: providing a systematic way of determining promotions, transfer, salary increases.

2. **Informative**: making available data to management on performance of subordinates, and to individuals on their strengths and weaknesses.

3. **Motivational**: creating a learning experience for subordinates that motivates them to improve.

If staff-related PIs are used in isolation, these can remain ineffective as an organisational measure. On the other hand, if these indicators are considered with measures related to, for example, teaching methods, unit costs, value-added, learning environment and so on, then we have a comprehensive set of PIs which promises to provide an effective measure of organisational performance. Without an effective system, no organisation can operate effectively. There is much evidence to suggest that not only does a poor human system cause organisational ineffectiveness, it can be destructive to the people who live and work in it (Porter *et al.*, 1975).

Teaching Methods

Documentation of teaching effectiveness in nurse education is essential to demonstrate the institution's accountability to the resource providers, professional bodies, and the public it serves. PIs related to teaching methods are useful measures of teaching effectiveness. PIs outlined below can be used for evaluating teaching methods in Nurse/Midwifery/Health Courses.

Teaching Methods

Indicators

- opportunities and support given to staff to experiment in different teaching styles.
- a variety of teaching skills is determined by all teaching staff.
- the introduction of new and relevant teaching skills is evident.
- contract learning and team teaching is practised where appropriate.
- the variety of teaching styles is adequately resourced.
- teaching is research-based.
- staff are involved in curriculum development.

Teaching effectiveness must also be demonstrated in clinical effectiveness. Clinical effectiveness is the teacher's ability to help students to transfer classroom learning to practice. To measure the effectiveness of clinical teaching, the following factors can be taken as indicators:

Indicators of Clinical Teaching Effectiveness

1. Teacher's knowledge
2. Clinical competence
3. Clinical supervision
4. Enthusiasm/stimulation
5. Effectiveness of teachers
6. Group instructional skill

These can be measured in various ways: instructor knowledge, clinical competence, and clinical supervision from personnel records and working schedules; enthusiasm/stimulation from observation of student/teacher interactions; and teachers' effectiveness and group instructional skill from student feedback.

Learning Environment

There is a close relationship between learning environment and learning effectiveness. A good learning environment is one that demonstrates good teaching, sensitive assessment methods, openness to students, and an approach which allows higher cognitive levels to be developed. A good learning environment sets the conditions for a desire to learn, a favourable attitude to study, and understanding of fundamentals.

Performance indicators for the learning environment can be divided into two areas in educational institutions where healthcare courses are provided: the ward/placement (clinical) and the college (classroom) environment. The following are relevant for evaluating the effectiveness of the learning environment.

Learning Environment	
Input:	Faculty/Department/Centres Funding Support services Organisational structure.
Process:	Setting and facilities Climate Teacher–student interaction.
Outcomes:	Accreditation Audits Placements.

It is imperative that the above indicators are applied with care and managed sensitively. As a priority, faculty and administrative support must be activated. Workshop or group sessions provide useful areas for considering and exploring staff concerns. A realistic timetable that considers the impact of change on faculty/department and administration has to be developed. Furthermore, sensitivity to faculty/departmental resistance and administrative constraints is imperative. Ideally, the new system should be phased in over time rather than imposed arbitrarily. The case study below demonstrate these considerations.

Case study: The faculty of nursing at a particular institution was able to introduce successfully PIs related to learning because of the sound and sensitive approach adopted. The faculty provided support and necessary information to the developers of PIs related to the learning environment. The Head of Faculty played a key role in setting up a task group to develop this initiative. She encouraged the faculty staff to participate in the field-testing of instruments designed by this group. Because of the greater participation by the faculty, the application of these PIs was fully accepted, and all staff were keen to participate in the evaluation of the learning environment.

Clinical Learning Environment

In nurse education the learning climate is not just confined to the classroom, but extends to clinical areas as well. It is imperative that various aspects of clinical teaching are evaluated. Research studies suggest that clinical placements do not always provide suitable learning environments for students (Fretwell,1980 and Orton, 1981). This highlights the necessity for the development of PIs for evaluating the effectiveness of the clinical learning environment. The following indicators suggest the existence of a good clinical learning environment:

- Profiles of the placement
- Established audit tools
- Regular auditing
- Review of completed audits undertaken by senior educationalists and managers
- Decisions regarding the suitability of a placement as a learning area are taken and communicated to those concerned.

Institutions which provide caring courses can develop very specific tools for auditing placement areas.

Peer Evaluation

Peer evaluation is a way forward in applying educational PIs related to the evaluation of learning environments. There is evidence to suggest that peer evaluation involving teaching and clinical (ward) staff will improve the clinical learning environment (Merchant, 1988). This joint venture will help bridge the gap between theory and practice that is experienced by many students.

Nicklin and Kenworthy (1987, p. 249) support the use of peer evaluation of their institution by staff from another teaching organisation for the following reasons:

> "…we believe there has previously been a 'them and us' mentality towards evaluation in nurse education, with a tendency for schools to maximise their strengths and minimise, if not conceal, their deficiencies. The inclusion of an independent evaluator provides the potential not only for a more open system of audit, but also for the transmission of good practices from one school to another"

Strategies which involve clinical nurses in the educational and evaluational processes are useful means by which the gap between theory and practice can be avoided. This can be achieved through discussion at ward level and use of questionnaires, both of which provide feedback.

Student Perception

The performance of a course or academic department is best assessed by finding out how effectively its students learn. The student perception procedure is one method of achieving this through use of a combination of interviews and questionnaires. The students' perceptions of the academic department and the approach they take to learning tasks are closely related. The student perception method places the focus on learning rather than teaching, and this is particularly useful where learning is seen as more than just enabling student to memorise formulae or trot out received opinion. There has been a fundamental shift in nurse education from such a method, and the student perception technique is a starting point in ascertaining its effectiveness. It is possible to define eight areas which students use to describe the characteristic of the academic departments which affect their learning (Ramsden, 1980).

The Eight Scales Dimensions of the Learning Environment

Relationship	Closeness of lecture/student relationships; help and understanding shown to students.
Commitment to teaching	Commitment of staff to improving teaching to students at a level appropriate to their current understanding.
Workload	Pressure placed on students in terms of demands of the syllabus and assessment tasks.
Formal teaching	Formality or informality of teaching (e.g. lecture or individual tuition).
Vocational	Perceived relevance of courses to students' careers; frequency and quality of academic and social relationship between students.
Clear goals	Extent to which standards expected of students are clear and unambiguous.
Freedom in Learning	Amount of discretion possessed by students in choosing and organising academic work.
Social Climate	Supportive learning environment.

Ramsden (1980) p. 139

33

Qualitative Aspects

The use of student perception techniques allows a better interpretation of what we mean by a 'good learning environment'. I would like to introduce you to Ramsden's (1980) findings to illustrate the value of the student perception procedure. Ramsden found the heavy workload in the applied science department was more readily acceptable than the much lighter one in the social science department. The arts and social science undergraduates resented formal teaching, whereas the science students thought that this was necessary. Ramsden writes:

> "What the science students meant by a good teaching relationship was different from what the arts student meant. The differences seem to be empirical remainders of the uncontroversial statement (often forgotten by traditional course evaluation) that what is a 'good' learning environment for students in one department or subject area is not necessarily good in another"

Ramsden, 1980, p. 140

I have indicated the reasons for the use of the student perception technique, and I have also outlined what I mean by a good learning environment. The student perception technique as a performance measure offers an opportunity to evaluate the effectiveness of the learning environment from a learning point of view.

Student review

Students are the best judges of teaching effectiveness and they can give valid and reliable answers based on their observation of a teacher's performance. Findings from student reviews of teaching effectiveness can be used as a diagnostic feedback to the teacher and as one of several sources of information. There is evidence to suggest that teachers who receive favourable ratings from students promote higher levels of student achievements on objective tests than teacher receiving less favourable ratings (Murray, 1984). This obviously suggests some correlation between high-quality outputs.

However, there are some disadvantages in the use of student reviews:

1. Local adaptation, i.e. student reviews need to be adapted and tailored to reflect a particular course programme; for example, a two-level evaluation tool which includes core items used in all functional departments of the college together with optional items developed by individual departments and faculty members.

2. Student reviews as universal indicators can make teachers suspicious of evaluation of their teaching. As I said earlier, work has to be undertaken to make these acceptable as PIs (see Chapter Two).

3. It is easy to establish that student review mechanisms have been set up. It is much more difficult to establish that they are being used effectively.

In the main, student reviews are beneficial as PIs to institutions, provided local validation of the rating instruments are carried out and the validity is ascertained before an instrument is used for policy decisions.

Questionnaires

The questionnaire format of student reviews lends itself well to development of PIs related to teaching effectiveness. Questionnaires are easy to handle, i.e. data can be collected quickly, efficiently and cheaply. Analysis of data is easy and findings can be quickly reported. Pilot questionnaires can be used to test for validity and reliability of performance indicators.

Student review of teaching effectiveness may include the following:

- Teaching methods
- Fairness, which primarily concerns assessment/testing
- Interest in me (student).

Global questions may be asked such as "how would you rate the teacher in comparison with all others that you had up until now?"

Other question for both students and teachers may concern:

a) course organisation;
b) selection of content;
c) relevance of content to the continuity of the course sequence; and
d) the relevance and quality of the course syllabus and related materials.

SUMMARY

The focus in this chapter has been on the application of PIs related to management and organisation, staff performance, teaching methods and the learning environment. The value of student reports, reviews and perceptions, and peer reviews has been considered and justified as fundamental to the evaluation process of an educational institution. The following are considered in the next chapter: the application of PIs related to unit costs; student-staff ratio (SSR); wastage and completion rates; value-added and examination/assessment results, as well as the strategies for introducing PIs in an educational institution.

Further Activities

1. Using the eclectic approach suggested in Chapter 3, develop indicators for the following aspects of organisational performance:

   Management & Organisation
   Staff Performance
   Learning Environment.

2. How would you ensure that student reports are objective?

3. Design a questionnaire for student review of teaching effectiveness.

Chapter Five:
Quantitative Factors in Nurse Education

The focus of this chapter is on calculable indicators such as unit costs, student-staff ratio (SSR), wastage and completion rates, value-added and examination/assessment results. These indicators should be used in conjunction with the qualitative ones described in Chapter Four to give an overall picture of the effectiveness of an educational institution such as a college of nursing, midwifery and health studies.

Unit Cost

Unit cost is a general measure given by the expression:

$$\frac{\text{Total Costs}}{\text{Number of Units}}$$

The use of unit costs as PIs will allow institutions to show how they use their resources in an effective and efficient way, and at the same time maintain quality. In nurse education, the most important 'units' are students, so an important unit cost is 'cost per student'. Financial managers of teaching establishments may use the simple 'cost per student' as a PI to demonstrate the effectiveness of their use of resources. However, this approach should be adopted with caution. Many studies have concentrated on unit costs as tools of comparison without paying enough attention to the many factors contributing to unit costs. Taking this point into account, the CIFPA (1988) states:

> "The concept of unit cost is relatively easy to understand but must be considered alongside the underlying factors which influence costs. This type of indicator is therefore at its most effective when used in conjunction with other indicators and information, e.g. about socio-economic factors"

> p. 13

It is important that firm conclusions are not drawn from unit cost measurements in isolation. It is tempting, for example, to assume that the lower the unit cost, the greater the efficiency. This assumption could well be false, since we may be ignoring or failing to take into full account many important factors which have a bearing on the result. This was pointed out by Burnip *et al.* (1980, p 73).

Quantitative Factors

If a cost measure such as the staff-student ratio (described below) is the **only** cost unit, it ignores all inputs other than the labour supplied by teachers. There is a danger that this may encourage the inefficient substitution of other inputs (for example, equipment, or secretarial or administrator time) for inputs from lecturers. Also, in this simple approach there is no attempt to make the distinction between teachers of different seniority and income levels. This may lead to distorted measurement and distorted incentives.

Further difficulties may be encountered in using cost measures as PIs (Cave *et al.*, 1988). For example, there may be a problem of conflicting interpretations of high cost per student because of uncertainty about output quality. By one interpretation, a high unit cost (say a high staff-student ratio) may be taken as an indicator of a high-quality education process. However, it is difficult to make this assumption in educational institutions such as College of Nursing where it has not always customary to make classified awards (graduation certificates).

We have to be sure that the bases used for the calculation and the assumptions made are comparable. Cost effectiveness comparisons between institutions would be straightforward if each had access to the same production technologies and faced identical prices. However, this is rarely the case. For example, different teaching institutions are likely to be using different educational technologies (computer facilities, software) with different price tags.

In spite of these difficulties, unit costs have a place in colleges. Unit costs can highlight the relationship between quality of teaching and student achievements, and enable one college to be compared with another in terms of cost efficiency. All colleges have to justify their costs, and unit costing is one method of enabling them to do so.

Student-Staff Ratio

The crude student-staff ratio used in some colleges, is simply the number of students divided by the number of teaching staff. The SSR defined by the Councils and Education Press (1972) is a valuable PI and has been used successfully in the public sector. The Councils and Education Press define SSR as follows:

If S =   the FTE (Full-time equivalent) no. of students;

     T =   the FTE no. of teachers;

     ACS =   the 'Average Class Size';

     ALH =   the 'Average Lecture Hours'
                      (i.e. the typical teaching hours of a FTE teacher)

ASH = the 'Average Student Hours'
(i.e. the typical taught hours of FTE students)

Then the teaching establishment required by a College is given by:

$$T = \frac{S}{ACS} \times ASH \times \frac{1}{ALH}$$

and the student/staff ratio by:

$$SSR = \frac{ACS \times ALH}{ASH}$$

Colleges must be able to justify their resources, and SSR, as defined above, can be used by managers of nurse education to ensure that resources are obtained and used efficiently in the accomplishment of the organisation's goal. SSR is useful as a tool for management but it must not be used in isolation. It must be combined with units to measure the effectiveness of education (quality of learning and so on). SSRs as PIs are useful in ensuring that colleges achieve the best possible economic return.

Economic return

What we mean by obtaining the best economic return is the achievement of the optimal relationship between expenditure and outcome (return), whereas the related term 'thrift' means simply the avoidance of expenditure which is not strictly necessary, or not necessary at the particular level (Kronig, 1978)

Wastage and Completion Rates

Wastage (i.e. the number of course leavers before completion date) and completion rates (i.e. the number of students completing the course) can be used as indicators of the quality of teaching. The findings from these indicators would be of considerable use for planning purposes, especially in courses where an attempt is made at planning labour supply, as well as in monitoring the success of an institution in producing qualified staff. The value of these measures lies in the way in which they are used. If they are used sensitively and in conjunction with other indicators such as entry standard, cost per student etc., they can be valuable in revealing possible problems within the institutions. For example, a higher education institution which combined high wastage rates, with higher entry standards, high costs, and a low publication rate could be deemed to have problems.

A high wastage rate indicates the need for investigations into causes. A higher level of wastage, for example, as a result of the standards on the course would be due to poor initial selection. Furthermore, it would be pertinent to distinguish between compulsory and voluntary wastage. It is possible that there might be different reasons for each, and in regard to voluntary wastage, the relevant performance indicators could be formulated to incorporate an evaluation of the procedures for counselling students.

Finally, PIs relating to attrition need to be developed to measure the effectiveness of support services as well for college students, and there may be found to be a relationship between wastage and quality of education.

Value-added Scores

The value-added scores can be useful in the measurement of institutional efficiency. They can be used to measure the effectiveness of transfer of knowledge from an 'educated' person to a 'less educated' person, as manifested by an increase in the productivity of the 'less educated' person. Cave *et al.* (1988) explain the concept of value-added:

> "The concept of value-added is simple. We consider two
> individuals identical in every respect until the decision
> to enter higher education is taken. One goes on to take a
> degree of a given quality; the other does not. The value
> added by the degree is the difference in the contribution
> made to the welfare of a society by the two individuals"

p. 59

It can be deduced from this definition that the more efficient institution produces much more value-added at the same or a lower cost. It follows that the efficiency of one institution relative to any other can be crudely measured by the rates of average value-added to average cost. Therefore, the higher the ratio, the more efficient the institution would be.

There is evidence to suggest that the introduction of value-added programme can be beneficial. Taylor (1985) claims that there were important benefits from this programme at a particular institution. Firstly, the faculties within that institution started taking the view that 'students come first'. The emphasis had shifted from attention given to quality alone to attention being given to both quantity and quality. Secondly, it has allowed the institution to demonstrate to funding authorities and to the general public that the education process is contributing value to individuals. This allows it to claim with justification that resources devoted to educating the students were well invested.

Value-added can be measured in a number of ways, and these include attitude surveys, interviews, objective standard tests, course taking patterns, subjective testing and extensive performance sampling of qualified nurses at various stages after completion of courses. An example would be the impact of well-qualified nurse/midwife teachers on less-qualified teachers under their supervision, or the impact of their role as mentors to other teachers.

Examination/Assessment Results

Test scores/examination results can be a useful measure of effectiveness of educational institution if used sensibly, because they are comparable, quantitative, and concise. They must be used along with other PIs suggested earlier to give a true picture of a particular institution's performance. Extreme care is needed when using examination/assessment results in comparing colleges' performance. Care must be taken to ensure that the information provided is fair and meaningful and can be accurately interpreted. Similar care must be taken to ensure that all figures used from examination boards are comparable, and that any comparisons are presented in a standardised format.

This chapter has introduced some useful ideas related to PIs for colleges. These include Unit Costs, Student Staff Ratio (SSR), Wastage Rates, Value-added Score, and Examination/Assessment results. Also, the value of all these measures and the contexts in which education institutions can apply them have been demonstrated. The next chapter outlines the strategies that you may adopt to develop these PIs for your institution.

Activities

1. Calculate the SSR for your college using the formula on page 34.

2. (a) To what extent are value-added scores used in nurse education?

   (b) How beneficial are these as PIs?

3. What reservations would you have about the use of examination/assessment results as measures of educational effectiveness?

4. Are any similar measures used in your establishment? How do they compare with the measures covered in activities 13 above.

Chapter Six:
Strategies for Introducing
Performance Indicators

Case Illustration

Mary Green, the Principal of New College, has delegated the responsibility for developing and implementing performance indicators for the college to the Vice-Principal, Bill Baker. Bill realises that his choice of methods for developing the measures and introducing them to the establishment will determine the success or otherwise of their implementation.

Activity: What strategies can Bill adopt to ensure the successful introduction of performance indicators into New College?

Many managers, like Bill, are faced with similar challenges. Implementing PIs in a large organisation can be a difficult task, but with the appropriate strategies for introducing change, the transition can be a smooth one for everybody. An outline of the necessary strategies of management that you as a manager can adopt in introducing PIs for your institution is provided below.

Strategy 1 – Create Ownership and Involvement
This is paramount for successful innovation and change. Involve the users in the changes related to PIs at an early stage. In the jargon, get the stakeholders (staff) to 'own' the changes. Ownership of the proposed developments will give you the staff's support because they have a hand in them from the start.

Strategy 2 – Create a positive Environment for Change
This means that you must adopt the following approach:
- be positive about the changes
- listen and respond to users
- sensitively support people involved in the development
- be open about problems and solutions
- encourage questioning and initiative
- reduce as much as you can the negative forces of factors militating against change, such as limited resources, constraints, negative attitudes, etc.

- utilise positive forces for change
- concentrate on people as resources and as having the power to influence and accept the development.

Strategy 3 – Identify the Needs for Change with Stakeholders/Users

Involve the members of your Management Team, Curriculum Development Teams and other key people in recognising the need for measures of performance. Influence the stakeholders, who are full of opinions, to contribute in the recognition of problems and the identification of remedies.

Assess the following sources in arriving at a managerial diagnosis of problems:

- past management problems
- past curriculum
- meetings
- observations of teaching and clinical activities
- talking and listening to other staff and students
- evaluation feedbacks.

Make a reflective record of all the above activities and this will provide you with useful information for making a diagnosis and planning an action of change.

Strategy 4 – Work out with your management team and staff (Audit group) an action plan for implementing your programme of organisation performance

This may include:

a) team development of some of the organisational measures;

b) a team-designed model for PIs; and

c) a requirement for all members of team to communicate the developments related to PIs to all others directly involved in nurse education.

Strategy 5 – Establish Personal Contacts

It is highly desirable that you establish contacts with key personnel in your organisation. They will open up your access to other people and openly support and disseminate your ideas of change. This approach will enhance your credibility and reputation and help you gain the influence and support for your programme of change.

Strategy 6 – Communicate the changes/developments.

Communicate your complex ideas in a simple way, and try to gain access, if you can, to formal/informal meetings and all in-service/continuing education programmes to sell your ideas of change, but be warned—there may be challenges or lack of understanding. Persevere professionally with your ideas and stick to your reasons as to why changes are needed. Talk to as many students as possible: as customers, their contribution will be valuable for testing your ideas relating to developments you are going to introduce.

Engage your interpersonal skills in full by:

- communicating plainly: transmit facts, ideas and feelings to others;
- listening: take time to hear and understand others' views;
- being an advocate: be able to reason out and justify ideas or courses of action;
- leading and motivating others;
- being able to evaluate and criticise contributions of others in a manner which encourages rather than threatens them;
- being able to accept criticism from others without being over-defensive.

Finally, put into use your image as a trustworthy, credible and appealing person. It will work wonders for the developments you are going to bring about.

Strategy 7 – Beware of Conflicts and Resistance
Get to know why people resist. Reasons may include:

- uncertainty about the development
- lack of knowledge and skills regarding the content of the change or how to implement it;
- lack of confidence;
- loss of influence and power;
- resentment of implied criticism of present practice;
- concerns about perceived increase in work load.

Openness and flexibility on your part will encourage questioning, initiative and expression of difficulties. Listening may provide opportunities for expression of pent-up emotional feelings. Release of emotions may affect responses to change in a positive way.

Utilisation of other strategies such as providing support, creation of positive environment, etc. may reduce conflicts and resistances. Also, do recognise that conflicts have a positive effect in requiring you to justify changes for sound reasons—not all changes are justifiable!

Strategy 8 – Encourage and foster the formation of Support Group Meetings.

For example, a 'managing change in education' support group for teaching and clinical staff could be set up to explore difficulties and solutions. Appoint facilitators to enable the following:

- creation of group trust and cohesiveness;
- the group to become 'change agents' and 'disciples' of change;
- the group to formulate an action plan to assist with changes; and
- group to hold follow-up meetings to share progress of change in terms of their action plan.

The above strategies have been found workable by many managers who have faced the task of introducing change. Do not be put off by initial resistance to developments. Persevere—it will be worth while in the end.

Finally, I outline below some reference works you may like to read before starting on your task.

The values of a positive environment as one of the recipes for managing change are well documented in management and allied literature. They include studies on organisational health (Miles, 1965); positive ethos (Everard and Morris, 1985: Elliot Kemp, 1982); and supportive climate (Fox, *et al.*, 1964; Sieber, 1968 and Fretwell, 1985).

The creation of ownership and the involvement of stakeholders aids and abets the management process of change. The managerial emphasis on ownership of innovations and involvement of stakeholders is found in the following literature: Fullen *et al.* (1985); Fretwell (1985) and Pratt (1980).

There should be managerial emphasis for the need for appropriate channels of communication to inform all concerned with the developments. The need for open, clear and uncomplicated communication is stressed by Elliot-Kemp (1982) Everard *et al.*, (1985), Fretwell (1985), Bevis (1978) Fullan *et al.* (1981) and Collister (1984), *inter alia.*

Support groups play a complementary role in enabling the developments to take place smoothly and they certainly reduce conflicts and resistance against change. The values of support groups are stressed by Fretwell (1985) and Bevis (1979). Furthermore, openness and flexibility help in the management of conflicts and resistance. A conceptual awareness of the causes of conflicts and resistance provides a useful guide in regard to the adoption of appropriate strategy of change (Handy, 1985; ENB, 1987 and Docking, 1987).

Chapter Seven:
Putting PIs Into Action

In the previous two chapters, I have given a description and some examples of PIs related to colleges. I have also given the reasons for their use. We now turn to some guidance on the procedures and processes of implementing a system of PIs related to Nurse/Midwifery and Health Studies.

First and foremost, a clear protocol is necessary so that all users and participants are aware of the system you are going to use. The PIs/audit mechanism must be user-friendly, otherwise all your efforts will be undermined because of the system's ineffectiveness. I suggested earlier in Chapter One, pilot testing of the scheme may prove to be useful in rendering the whole process effective later.

A user-friendly guide may also prove useful for users and participants. An example of an academic audit guide is provided for you on the next few pages.

AUDIT GUIDE

What is an academic audit?

An academic audit provides the opportunity to monitor the process of education against a set of criteria-based standards. The focus of this audit is on the Project 2000 Course.

It encompasses a systematic data collection, evaluation, analysis and written report of performance of the course. Performance evaluation in education, carried through the academic audit, embraces:

- all aspect of the activities within the programme under review.
- consideration of the effectiveness, i.e., quality, the relationship between expectations and outcomes.

An educational programme can be said to provide a quality service and value for money if the audit process shows that it is achieving educational objectives effectively and efficiently.

How is the audit process carried out ?

As a guide rather then a blueprint, the following sequence for carrying the audit process is suggested:

1. Establish audit team (see section on who are the auditors).

2. Issue information about the exercise to all those who need to know/be involved.

3. Get agreement to proceed with the audit.

4. Collect data using the audit instrument provided.

5. Record data on audit mechanism.

6. Make essential judgement by applying agreed criteria to data collected.

7. Produce a written report of findings with recommendations for action.

8. Devise an Action Plan in consultation with relevant parties.

9. Send Action Plan and Summary to Audit Team.

10. Audit team notify the audit report to the Quality Assurance Manager.

Who are the Auditors?

The concept of an audit embraces a critical and objective examination of an educational programme, ideally undertaken by skilled and experienced personnel who traditionally have been impartial and without personal bias. The auditors lack of self-interest have endowed their unbiased investigation and subsequent report with credibility and reliability. To keep-up with the spirit of this claim, we recommend that the following personnel should carry out the audit.

Course Managers (Heads of CFP and Branch programmes), peers from another college, and clinical colleagues should comprise the audit team for the purpose of auditing the course.

What is being audited?

The purpose of an academic audit is to review the quality of the services provided within the course. The ultimate aim of the audit is concerned with confirming and reporting current practices, and offering positive recommendations to secure improved performance.

Both qualitative and quantitative data will be acceptable evidence on which the auditors will base their judgements.

What is the academic audit form?

The form is a set of audit statements designed for use by auditors as an instrument to obtain data relevant to review the educational programme in terms of quality.

The audit form has been designed as a working document for the purpose of academic audit. It is not intended as an exhaustive or comprehensive tool but to provide the crucial starting point in the continuing process of reflection, analysis and evaluation. It is anticipated that the audit form provides positive encouragement to intending users to appreciate that the guiding principles in conducting sound audits are common sense and inquisitiveness.

It is generally accepted that there are no ideal measures nor universally applicable indicators of excellence in educational auditing.

Each main question found in the audit form is followed by sub-questions and each of these is related to specific performance indicators (see page 54).

How to use the audit questionnaire? The audit form should not be seen as prescriptive or restrictive. The form provides a common language and is user-friendly.

The following make-up the academic audit form:

1. Statement and sub-statement with a section for "YES" or "NO" response and a space for comments.

2. Action plan and summary sheet.

Auditors are required to check that each question related to the main statement is achieved and then complete the value-judgement section. The action that is going to be taken must be indicated (see page 53).

The action plan and summary section must be completed in consultation with the appropriate course managers. The action plan and summary will be sent to the audit team. The audit team will send a report of the findings to the Senior Management Team.

PROJECT 2000 COURSE AUDIT TEAM.

Format for implementing Performance Indicators (PIs)

I cannot tell you exactly what your PIs should be, but they must be **relevant, accurate** and **feasible** (see Chapter 2).

What options do we have for physically collecting the important data we need? The questionnaire format has proved the most suitable one for many institutional measures related to performance. An example is provided below:

Basic Course Information

Please give figures relating to the last 12 months

		Adult	Mental	Learning Disab- ilities	Children
Bursary Students					
Salaried Students					
Number of Intakes/Year					
Wastage Rates (%)	1st Year				
	2nd Year				
	3rd Year				
Examination Results	1st Entry				
	2nd Entry				
No. & % of Passes	3rd Entry				
Student/Teacher Ratio					

For more complex data, I suggest a format adapted from the work of Further Education Unit (FEU, 1989): *"Towards an Educational Unit"*. You need the following: a lead sheet, a continuation sheet, an action plan, and a summary sheet.

The lead sheet

The lead sheet identifies the broad area of the audit exercise, giving indicators of the purpose(s) of audit, details of the audit team and the data on reference to available audit instruments, PIs and other relevant documentation which is both illustrative of approaches to similar exercises developed and trial-tested at other educational institutions. Figure 6 below shows the proposed layout for the lead sheet of the audit questionnaire package.

FIGURE 6: Example Lead sheet

Educational Audit

Date: **Undertaken By:**

Topic Area:

STATEMENT	Primary Reason For Audit
Teaching Methods Are courses evaluated for effectiveness in terms of teaching methods?	☐ On-going review ☑ Quality improvement ☐ Report to external agency ☐ Institutional renewal ☐ Efficiency improvement ☐ Health and Safety ☐ Other:

---

adapted from FEU (1990) p. 6

Figures 7 & 8 below shows the proposed layouts of the continuation and action sheets.

Figure 7: Continuation Sheet

EDUCATIONAL AUDIT

  DATE: **UNDERTAKEN BY:**
  TOPIC AREA:

Audit Question	Performance Indicators	Value Judgement		Action
		Satisfactory Yes/No	Criteria of satisfaction/ Further attention	

Figure 8: Action Plan

EDUCATIONAL AUDIT: ACTION PLAN

Topic Area: Teaching Effectiveness
Action By:Position: **Date:**

Description of action to be undertaken	Person Responsible	Time Allocated	Comp. Date	Resources Required	Antici- pated Benefits
Obtain reviewed profile of teacher's qualifications	Head of CFP	2 weeks	10 Oct 1992		Planning staff develpt. prog.
Establish register of all research undertaken by staff	Heads of Studies	8 weeks	14 Nov 1992		Extent of research effort

Summary Sheet

Figure 9 below shows the proposed layout for a summary sheet.

Figure 9: Summary Sheet

EDUCATIONAL AUDIT SUMMARY SHEET
Started: **Completed:**   **Undertaken by:**
EVALUATION OF AUDIT EXERCISE
Timeliness: Was the audit undertaken at the appropriate time? *Yes*
Clarity: Were the results clearly understandable? *Yes, by all concerned*
Activation: Did the results facilitate action? *Action areas identified and initiated*
Cost: Details of actual cost: hours, resources, consumables. etc. *4 staff hours + working lunch*
Effectiveness: Intended/Potential benefits *1.   Improvement in quality* *2.   Course development*
Comments on Audit Process: Negotiation, Involvement, Ownership, Commitment etc. *The involvement of staff with the Course Leader and* *Head of Faculty was particularly valuable.*
REPORT TO: *Principal*
RECOMMENDATIONS: *1. Monitor & produce a report of staff* *progress in relation to development* *programme.* *2. Produce faculty's profile of* *publications of research undertaken.*
Signed: **Date:**

Performance Indicators

Some examples of questions and PIs for Organisational audits are given below under various headings:

Mission Statement

Is there evidence of a clearly defined mission statement?

Question	Performance Indicators
Is there a statement of mission?	Published evidence of mission statement.
Who was involved in the formulation of mission statement? e.g. Principal, Senior Management; Academic Board; Academic Staff; Students.	Documentation/Notes of the process of evolution of mission statement. Documentation of the contributory activities of the participants.
Has the contribution of participants reflected in the mission statement?	Records/notes/minutes of debate and recommendation of participants.
Is it widely understood?	Questionnaires; Staff handbook; Student handbook; Prospectus.
Is there evidence of ownership of mission statement?	Questionnaires; minutes of meetings; publicity material.
How is it validated? —externally —internally	Procedure established and documented in relation to both internal and external validation.
How frequently is the mission or purpose statement reviewed? — annually — 1–3 years — 3–10 years.	Review and evaluation documents of mission statement.
What areas are addressed in mission statement? e.g. evaluation; training; equal opportunities; income generation; etc.	Mission statement details.
Are these areas addressed in the mission statement priorities?	

Organisational Structures

Is the present organisation structure appropriate to the strategic purpose of the Institution/Unit?

Question	Performance Indicators
What is the present structure?	Defined organisational chart.
What are the links with the statutory bodies/funding bodies?	—Defined relationships —Agreed planning cycles —Monitoring/reviews.
Is the organisation structure a reflection of organisation purpose?	—Mission statement —Academic/Faculty/Dept. plans —Regular Reviews —Date of last reorganisation.
Is there a documented procedure to support the organisation structure?	—Defined job descriptions —Infrastructure of plans, policies and operating manual.

Decision Taking And Information Systems

Has the institution/functional units a clear and effective system of decision making in which delegated authority is based at the lowest appropriate level and is supported by a comprehensive system of relevant and updated information?

Question	Performance Indicators
Is there a distinctive statement outlining areas of responsibility, lines of communication, and current operating procedures relating to the annual cycle of college activities?	—An updated operating procedure manual (indicating, e.g. relationships, responsibilities, systems, forms, deadlines. —regularly revised job descriptions.
Who has responsibility for maintaining the procedure?	—designated responsibility —loose leaf/word processor disk.
Has the institution/functional unit reviewed reallocation of decisions to lower levels within the organisation?	—Minutes of organisation review meeting —Revised job descriptions —Staff development reviews.
Is there greater staff participation in corporate activities?	—(as above)

Performance Indicators

Is decision-making based on statement policy and objectives?	Evidence of correlation.
Do decision-makers have access to the relevant information upon which to formulate decisions?	—Management Information System (MIS) relates to decision makers' needs and clear justification of decisions taken.
Are the results of decisions reported back to those responsible?	—Effective MIS
Do the institution's general policies, procedures and evidence of recent staff development provide support to improve decision making.	—Evidence of management training.
Has the institution adopted mechanisms and a culture which supports the reflection and analysis of past decisions?	—Dept./functional reviews —Regular staff reviews —Supportive counselling.
Is there wide and relevant participation in institutional decision processes?	Involvement of: —governors/management executives —advisory members —staff —students —clients.
Are management decisions minuted and disseminated to those affected?	—Minutes —Distribution —Meetings schedule.
Has the institution undertaken a needs analysis to identify essential management information requirements?	—Sampling of information provided and comments from management. —Extent of on-line facilities.
How does the institution/functional unit communicate the general awareness about the need for information from staff?	—Briefing meetings —Departmental meetings —Staff seminars.
How does the institution/functional unit ensure an adequate system of dissemination of information to staff.	—Meetings —Minutes —Newsletters —Participation.

56

| To what extent has the Institution adopted the new technologies in decision making and communication | —Use of on-line MIS
—Use of FAX
—Use of modern lines
—Use of new switchboard systems. |

Teaching Methods

Are courses evaluated for effectiveness in terms of teaching methods?

Questions	**Performance Indicators**
Are there opportunities and support for staff to use different teaching styles?	—staff development programme —student evaluation feedback
Is there evidence of a variety of teaching skills demonstrated by all teaching staff?	—as above —classroom visits. —peer review feedback
Is the introduction of new skills evident?	—as above
Is there evidence of contract learning and team teaching where relevant, being practised?	—documentation —peer review feedback.
Is the introduction of new skills evident?	—as above
Is there evidence of contract learning and team teaching, where relevant, being practised?	—documentation —peer review feedback.
Is there evidence to suggest that the variety of teaching styles are adequately resourced?	—availability and quality of teaching resources
Is teaching research-based?	—application of research findings.
Are teaching staff involved in curriculum development?	—minutes of meetings. —working records, etc.
What are the levels of teachers' professional and curriculum expertise?	—teachers' qualifications (proportions of graduates, etc.) —time devoted to management training for service staff. —proportion of staff with relevant recent INSET (In-Service Education and

	Training). —Use of College-based INSET and other studies. —Match of teaching programmes with the quality of such planning and schemes. —Staff appraisal scheme.
How effective is the management of learning process?	—Management and organisation of time and deployment of staff. —Teaching loads, management of hours and condition of service. —Student evaluation feedback of teaching effectiveness —Achievement of objectives —Assessment (diagnosis, feedback, remediation) —Reception and marking of work.
Is there evidence of quality relationship within the College?	—Effectiveness of communication between senior management and staff. —Delegated responsibility —Teamwork —Initiative —Students: discipline, sympathy, humour, awareness of individual, support.
What is the level of teaching staff dedication?	—industriousness —extra-curricular involvement. —attendance —punctuality —liaison with customers, care service providers and other establishments.
Is there evidence of student review of teaching effectiveness?	—student ratings —questionnaires —student evaluation feedback.
How effective is teaching?	—organisation/clarity of teaching programme

587864645345

53622222222

—enthusiasm/stimulation created by teachers
—clinical expertise/competence of practitioners
—level of student supervision
—quality of teaching by service/placement staff.

Learning Environment

How effective is the learning environment?

Questions	Performance Indicators
Are facilities appropriately funded?	—funding levels —budget statements.
Is there appropriate organisational structure?	—organisational charts.
Is climate suggestive of staff and student satisfaction?	—consumer/staff satisfaction survey questionnaires. —quality of staff/student interaction.
How effective is the clinical learning environment?	—availability of profiles of placement. —audit tools used —regularity of auditing —review of completed audits —decisions regarding suitability of placement as a learning area taken and communicated
Is there evidence of Peer evaluation of learning environment?	—Peer evaluation review feedback. Teamwork.
Is there evidence of use of student perception?	—Student Perception Inventory, data analysis and report.

Staff Performance

Academic Leadership

Are managers exercising appropriate leadership and ensuring that programmes are relevant to the demands of the market (caring and other services) they serve?

Questions

Performance Indicators

What is the need for academic leadership in the institution?

Record of outcome of course
—no. of new submissions
—no. of new developments introduced.
—nature of liaison with validating bodies.
—extent of staff development, e.g. courses completed; research/consultancy/ updating for Senior Staff.
—National/regional links and relationships
—Evidence of cost-effectiveness of development activity.

To what extent are institutional managers undertaking effective individual/team development?

—Course team development
—Subject specialist development
—Individual staff development
—Availability of managers to their teams
—Conscious activities to ensure high morale.

Academic and non-academic staff

Does the institution monitor, record and evaluate staff outcomes?

Question

Performance Indicators

Do all staff fulfil the class contact and other requirements to their agreed conditions of service?

—timetables
—SSR computations set against agreed targets and trends over a reasonable number of years
—Notional potential teaching hours vocational
—Verifications of under-time tabling and reasons.

Do all non-teaching staff fulfil their job requirements to their agreed conditions of service?

—workload and priorities
—organisation and completion of task as delegated.

Are there satisfactory procedures for assessing staff performance?

Records of staff meetings; interviews; counselling.

Are there provisions for staff development?	Staff development strategies statement; Staff development programme; records of INSET programmes; records of counselling meetings.
Is there evidence of staff development programmes?	Records of evaluation procedures and feedback. Questionnaires etc.
Are there mechanisms for monitoring, recording and reporting staff grievances?	Records
Do the staff grievance procedures allow for subsequent action?	Records; documentation of action.

Does the institution monitor, analyse and report on staff turn-over, absenteeism and punctuality?	MIS facilitating data on:
	i. staff turn-over
	ii. punctuality
	iii. staff absenteeism
	iv. comparative statistics
	      —locally
	      —regionally
	      —nationally
	      —internationally?

Are there mechanisms for identifying professional expertise within the institutions for external services?	Database of: —staff expertise —staff experience —projects —interest.
Are there procedures for exploring community needs expertise?	Institutional marketing strategy statement. Records of visits, meetings, conferences.
Are there procedures for exploring and analysing the community standing of the institution?	Questionnaire; polls; research projects.
Does the institution actively support staff initiatives in relation to external professional development?	Records of staff involvement in external services. Documentations of publishing procedures relating to staff achievements.
Does the institution monitor the cost of staff outcomes.	Calculation of costs per staff developed compared with agreed targets.

Academic Quality Assurance

Has the institution/functional unit a comprehensive system of academic planning linked to resource planning.

Question	Performance Indicators
Has the institution/functional unit a comprehensive system of academic planning?	Updated mission statement, strategic plans, academic plans, department plans.
What informs the planning mechanism?	Regional workforce planning departments requirements/ contracts. Up-to-date market intelligence: active marketing, employment trends; other advisory groups.
What is the system for initiating a new course?	Processes leading to submission to a course approvals panel of a detailed proposal for authorisation, e.g. Academic Board.
Is there a system of internal validation of course proposals prior to final validation procedures?	Internal faculty/college review group; Detailed check lists for validators; involvement of externals in system; Defined review groups; Specified operating procedures; Student, staff and employer questionnaires; Course team reviews.

Chapter Eight:
Conclusions

The early chapters of this book introduced several concepts related to performance indicators: definitions, theoretical models, processes by which measures of performance are applied, and several conceptual frameworks. The RCN's treatment of Donabedian's (1980) structure-process-outcome model is the approach most suitable for our purposes. The RCN has not only developed the Donabedian model adequately, but it offers examples of performance indicators for nurse education, and I demonstrated how these can be applied.

However, a theoretical understanding of performance indicators is not enough to allow their application as a tool for performance measurement. The **properties** of performance indicators are also important. Several authors have offered thoughts on these (Cave *et al.* 1988; Best 1983; Porter 1978)

Chapters 4 and 5 considered performance indicators (both subjective and objective) applicable in establishments of nurse education. The purpose and application was given for indicators related to management and organisation, staff performance, staff professional profile and student reporting. Examples of measures were given in the relevant sections, sufficient for you to work out a comprehensive set of performance indicators for your establishment.

Student reviews of teaching methods have hitherto been a much neglected notion in nurse education, and I would encourage you to use the examples provided in this book to construct student reviews as indicators of teaching effectiveness.

The gap between theory and practice is recognised as a serious problem in nurse education. Although indicators related to the learning environment are available in nurse education, there is scope for extensive use of peer evaluation involving teaching and clinical staff. Research evidence strongly suggests that peer evaluation will improve the clinical learning environment and help to narrow the gap between theory and practice (RCN, 1988).

Student perception can be used to assess how effectively an institution enable its students to learn. This concept is well developed and applied in higher education (Ramsden, 1980) but has been little used in nurse education. I would encourage also the use of student perception as a performance indicator for the learning environment.

Indicators related to staff performance, teaching methods and learning environment are fundamental to the evaluation of nurse education in terms of effectiveness and efficiency. Other indicators such as unit costs, student/staff ratio, wastage and completion rates, value-added and examination/assessment results are equally valuable. There is hardly any evidence of the application of these indicators in nurse education, although their application to schools and higher education establishments is well developed. Their use is recommended.

Concerns related to high wastage rates in nurse education strongly suggest that the concept of wastage and completion rates should be developed into performance indicators for measuring institutional performance.

Performance indicators in nurse education are often related to effectiveness in terms of its immediate end products, that is, the graduates of the College of Nursing. There is scope for developing value-added scores for the evaluation of these graduates. An argument was sustained for their development into performance indicators in nurse education in Chapter Five. There is a need to assess how well a qualified nurse may increase the productivity of less well qualified staff. Le Grand and Robinson (1979) and Cave et al. (1988) support this view in relation to university graduates, but suggest that it is equally applicable to nurse education and allied studies.

The evidence relating to indicators of examination results/test scores is relatively new to nurse education, although their usefulness is evident in schools (Gray et al., 1986). Their usefulness and pitfalls were highlighted in Chapter Five. There are means by which examination/assessment scores offer scope for development into indicators in comparing the performance of institutions.

The comprehensive set of performance indicators that you may have for your college must be matched by strategies for introducing them. Without these strategies it would not be easy for you to make the changes related to performance measures workable. Therefore, the eight strategies for introducing performance indicators considered in Chapter Six could act as a useful guide. These included creating ownership and involvement; creating a positive environment; identifying the needs for change with stakeholders/users; action plan for introducing PIs; establishing personal contacts; communicating the developments; managing conflicts and resistance; and fostering the formation of support group meetings.

A practical guide for audits related to PIs is provided in Chapter Seven. Readers are offered examples of a range of indicators of performance. There are opportunities for readers to adopt or develop their own indicators using the examples provided in this chapter.

In summary, therefore, although Colleges of Nursing have well-developed performance indicators related to staff performance, teaching methods and learning environment, they must look beyond these indicators in evaluating their effectiveness. Until concepts such as unit costs, SSRs, wastage and completion rates, value-added and examination results/scores are developed into performance indicators in nurse education institutions, colleges of nursing are not sufficiently evaluated to be able to demonstrate their effectiveness (Narayanasamy, 1991). The way forward for nurse education is to take on board the concepts and examples presented in this book and develop them along with existing measures to generate a more comprehensive set of indicators for colleges of nursing, midwifery and allied studies.

Glossary of Terms

Academic Audit	A procedure for monitoring the process of education against a set of criteria-based standards.
Criteria	Objective statements of the standard for comparison, against which performance can be measured.
Marketing	A process in which supply is matched with demand: i.e. having the right goods or services, of the right quality, in the right place, at the right time, and in the right amounts.
Measures	An instrument for measuring: i.e. ascertaining the quantity, quality, or dimension.
Mission Statement	A succinct expression of the purpose of an institution in terms of its goals and direction.
Model	A conceptual representation of a reality. It can be a symbolic or abstract representation of a real thing.
Organisation	An institution in which several staff are involved in providing a service to customers.
Peer Evaluation	A process of appraisal carried out by colleagues/fellow students.
Peer Review	An evaluation process carried out by colleagues/fellow workers/students.
Performance Indicators	Pointers which focus attention on many functions of an organisation which include resource use, quality of services, staff performance, support services, etc.
Reliability	The extent to which a measure or procedure produces similar results under constant conditions on all occasions.
Simple Indicators	Information presented as statistical data.
Stakeholders	Staff or others who have an interest or investment in an organisation related to, for example, services, goods, profits, careers, positions, status etc. Changes to the organisation almost inevitably affect its stakeholders.

Glossary

Standards

An agreed level of services required for a particular purpose. When standards are written, they should be reasonable, explicit, useful, measurable, observable, and achievable.

Student Perception

An evaluation process, usually of teachers, carried out from students' perspectives, e.g. Student Perception Inventory.

Student-Staff Ratio

The number of teaching staff to number of students, usually expressed as a ratio by dividing the number of students by the number of teachers. For example, the SSR is 1:20 where there is one teacher to twenty students.

Unit Cost

A component of any particular area of a unit expenditure that may have a financial implications, usually expressed in budgetary terms (financial statements).

Quality

Degree of excellence. For example, the characteristics of a quality educational service are efficiency, reliability, accessibility, value for money, student (consumer/customer) centred, high consumer satisfaction, etc.

Validity

Tells us whether an item measures or describes what it is supposed to measure or describe.

Value-added Scores

A measure that demonstrates how well an 'educated' person has contributed to the development of a 'less educated' person to become more efficient at work.

References

ANDERSON, R.G. *A Dictionary of Management Terms*. McDonald and Evans, 1983.

BEST, G. Performance Indicators: A precautionary tale for unit managers *In:* I. WICKINGS, ed. *Effective Unit Management*. King Edward Fund for London, 1983.

BETHEL, D. Indicators of Performance related to Students and Staff *In:* D. BILLING, ed. *Indicators of Performance*. Society for Research into Higher Education, 1980.

BEVIS, E.M.O. *Curriculum Building in Nursing*. St. Louis, USA: 1978.

BURNIP, M.S. and LINSELL, S. Indicators in Polytechnics *In:* K. DURANS and D. BILLING, eds. *Indicators of Performance*. Society for Research in Higher Education, 1980.

CAVE, M., HANNEY, S., KOGAN, M., and TRAVETT, G. *The Use of Performance Indicators in Education*. London: Jessica Kingsley, 1988.

CIPFA *Performance Indicators of Schools*. United Kingdom: Chartered Institute of Public Finance and Accountancy. 1988.

COLLISTER, B. Research into the process of attitude change and its implications for nurse education. *Nurse Education Today Journal*, 1984, 9296.

COUNCILS AND EDUCATION PRESS *Assessment of Curricular Education*. London: Councils and Education Press, 1972.

DONABEDIAN, A. *The Definition of quality and approaches to its assessment*. Michigan: Health Adminstration Press, 1980.

DOCKING, S. Curriculum innovation *In:* P. ALLAN and M. JOLLEY eds. *The Curriculum in Nurse Education*. London: Croom Helm, 1987.

ELLIOT-KEMP, J. *Managing Organisational Change: A Practitioner's Guide*. Sheffield: Sheffield City Polytechnic, Pavic Publications, 1982.

ENB *Managing Change in Nursing Education*. London: English National Board for Nursing, Midwifery and Health Visiting, 1987.

EVANS, L. Performance Indicators in Nurse Education. *Senior Nurse*, September 1987, **17**(3).

EVERARD, K.B. and MORRIS, G. *Effective School Management*. London: Harper & Row, 1985.

References

FEU *Towards an Educational Audit*. London; Further Education Unit (FEU), 1990

FRETWELL, J.E. Hospital ward routine—friend or foe? *Journal of Advanced Nursing*, 1981, 5(6), 625635.

FRETWELL, J.E. *Freedom to Change*. London: Royal College of Nursing, 1985.

FOX, R.S. and LIPPITT, R. The innovation of classroom mental health practices. *In:* M. MILES ed. *Innovation in Education*, New York: International Psychoanalytical Press, 1964.

FULLEN, M. and PARK, P. *Curriculum Implementation*. Ontario: The Ministry of Education, 1981.

GLASER, B. and STRAUSS, A. *The Discovery of Grounded Theory*. Chicago: Aldine Publishing Co., 1967.

GRAY, J., JESSON, D. and JONES, B. The search for a fairer way of comparing schools' examination results, *Research Papers in Education*, 1986, 1(2), 91121.

HANDY, C.B. *Understanding Organisations*, London: Penguin, 1985.

KERSHAW, B. and EVANS, L. Testing Skills, *Nursing Times*, 10 Dec 1986, 1920.

KRONIG, W. *Performance related budgeting for universities*, OECD/CERI IMHE/GC/78.7 paper for IMHE workshop on performance indicators for institutions of HE. Paris:1979.

LE GRAND, J. and ROBINSON, R. *The Economics of Social Problems*, London: MacMillan, 1979.

McGREGOR, D. *The Human Side of Enterprise*. New York: McGraw Hill, 1960.

MERCHANT J. Feedback methods in nursing education, *Nurse Education Today*, 1988, (8), 279283.

MILES, M. Planned change and organisation health. *In:* A. HARRIS, M. LAWN, and W. PRESSCOTT, eds., *Curriculum Innovation*. London: Croom Helm, 1975.

MURRAY, H. The impact of formative and summative evaluation of teaching in North American Universities. *Assessment and Evaluation in Higher Education*, 1984, 9(3), 117132.

NARAYANASAMY, A. The application of performance indicators to nurse education. Part 1 & 2, *Nurse Education Today*, 1991, (11), 335346.

NICKLIN, P. and KENWORTHY, N. Education Audit. *Senior Nurse*, July 1987, 7(1), 22–24.

ORTON, H.D. Ward learning climate and student response. *Nursing Times*. 1981, Occasional paper 77, 65–68.

PORTER, D. *Developing performance indicators for the teaching function*. Paper presented at the IMHE Fifth Special Topic workshop, June 1978, Paris [IMHE/GC/78.3].

PORTER, L.W., LAWLER, E.E. and HACKMAN, J.R. *Behaviour in Organisation*. New York: McGraw Hill, 1975

PRATT, J. Costing and Quality, *Higher Education Review*, 1979, (Summer).

RAMSDEN, P. Educating the quality of learning. *In:* D. BILLING, ed., *Indicators of Performance*: Society for Research in Higher Education. 1980

RCN *Performance Indicators in Nurse Education*. London: Royal College of Nursing, 1987 and 1988.

ROGUES, A. Cheers! *Nursing Times*, 27 January 1988, **84**(4), 1415.

SIEBER, S. D. Organizational influences on innovative roles *In:* D. EIDELT and L. KITCHELL, eds. *Knowledge Production and Utilisation*. University of Oregon, 1968.

SIZER, J. Assessing institutional performance: an overview. *International Journal of Institutional Management in Higher Education*, 1979, **3**(1), 4977.

SPROULL, L.S. and ZUBROW, D. Performance information in school systems: perspectives from organisational theory. *Education Adminstration Quarterly*, 1981

TAYLOR, T. A. Value-Added Student Model: North East Missouri State University, *Assessment and Evaluation in Higher Education*, 1985 **10**(3), 190202.

Index